CALISTHENICS

I0222725

The Ultimate Guide to Calisthenics for Beginners

(Get in Shape and Stay in Shape for the Rest of Your Life)

Lowell Aguayo

Published By Bella Frost

Lowell Aguayo

Calisthenics: The Ultimate Guide to Calisthenics for Beginners (Get in Shape and Stay in Shape for the Rest of Your Life)

ISBN 978-1-77485-241-5

Legal & Disclaimer

The information contained in this book is not designed to replace or take the place of any form of medicine or professional medical advice. The information in this book has been provided for educational and entertainment purposes only.

The information contained in this book has been compiled from sources deemed reliable, and it is accurate to the best of the Author's knowledge; however, the Author cannot guarantee its accuracy and validity and cannot be held liable for any errors or omissions. Changes are periodically made to this book. You must consult your doctor or get professional medical advice before using any of the suggested remedies, techniques, or information in this book.

Upon using the information contained in this book, you agree to hold harmless the Author from and against any damages, costs, and expenses, including any legal fees potentially resulting from the application of any of the information provided by this guide. This disclaimer applies to any damages or injury caused by the use and application, whether directly or indirectly, of any advice or information presented, whether for breach of contract, tort, negligence, personal injury, criminal intent, or under any other cause of action.

You agree to accept all risks of using the information presented inside this book. You need to consult a professional medical practitioner in order to ensure you are both able and healthy enough to participate in this program.

TABLE OF CONTENTS

Introduction

This book provides a step-by-step guide to begin the Calisthenics program. This book will get you given a brief introduction to calisthenics. You will learn the basics, what to expect, and things to think about (i.e. decide if it's the right fitness program) as well as the benefits and the motivation behind adopting the specific routine. Then, you're given the chance to comprehend the advantages for your wellbeing.

In addition In this book, you'll learn about various ways to carry out one of the most effective and practical exercises for calisthenics; A detailed explanation will be given to you. If you're looking to design your own calisthenics regimen You're now tutored by a professional and you'll receive instructions and even samples of exercises.

Chapter 1: Calisthenics 101

For Beginners

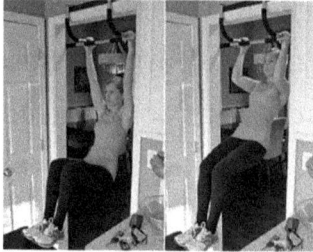

Albeit relatively new--in terms of gaining popularity--calisthenics are not new. Actually, the word originated from Greek word kalos (kallos) as well as thenos (sthenos). Kalos means beauty and emphasises the aesthetic pleasure that contributes to the perfect human physique. Sthenos is a synonym for strength and emphasizes mental as well as physically strong, courageous and determination. Calisthenics get names from Greek historian Callisthenes who was one of its first advocates. What do you know about Calisthenics?

Calisthenics refers to making use of the weight of your body to exercise your body, and develop an attractive physique that speaks volumes about the physical as well as mental power as well as the courage.

Calisthenics are an exercise that involves many gross motor movements like running, pushing and standing, grasping and other similar movements without the assistance of gym equipment, such as dumbbells or other equipment and are often performed in a rhythmic manner.

The fundamental concept behind Calisthenics is that it is an form of body-weight exercise that, by gross motor movements, aims to build your endurance, strengthen and build your muscles by using the natural motions like pushing as well as jumping.

When you make use of your body as a resistance device when you push, pull to bend, jump and swing you are increasing your strength and fitness as you perform the exercises with vigor and vigorously, you will improve your aerobic and muscular conditioning and psychomotor skills like coordination, balance, as well as agility.

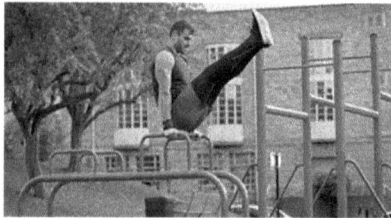

In the next section Let's examine how beneficial these kinds of exercises can be, especially when you consider the common belief of building muscle and sculpting the body is that it must be done with gym equipment.

The Benefits Of Calisthenics Exercises

If you've been reading the weight loss blogs and other publications and blogs, you'll notice that calisthenics have become extremely well-known. This type of exercise has been in practice for quite a long time, we are talking from the stone age in which man used to play the pull and push game, and other heavy objects and utilize his body to lift himself up trees while searching for fruit--you might be asking "what's the fuss about? Does the workout really have the same benefits as various Medias claim it as being?" The answer is that calisthenics can be wildly beneficial. In this article we will examine how beneficial this kind of exercise can be:

1: The No Need for Equipment

Although calisthenics is the practice of using weights that train the body using various gross motor abilities, some exercises based on calisthenics require the use of equipment like the pull-up bar or dumbbells. But should you be able to locate something that you can do pull-ups with then that's all you require. For illustration consider a sturdy door frame you can grasp (if there's enough room) or connect a pull up bar you can purchase on websites like Amazon at a price of less than $50 (check the image below)

If you think about the price of an exercise membership (often between $40 and $50 per month) and then look at the price of a pull-up bar, which, surprisingly, is the minimum you will need to perform calisthenics workouts The latter is a great way to save money.

Additionally, because you are able to utilize the pull-up bar from home, you can eliminate the requirement to convince yourself to get to the gym after an exhausting day at work If we're being truthful, is one of the main reasons that people do not exercise. This saves you both time and cash. Additionally, if you can't afford the 20 dollars or more it costs to buy a pull-up bar that you can put at home, you could go to a playground in the community and utilize your monkey bars (check the image below).

This adds a touch of fun to exercise and can break up the monotony that comes with weight training at a gym. This reduces the likelihood that you will become bored and stop working out.

2: The Full Body Training Aspect

Alongside targeting specific muscles, a significant part of the calisthenics workouts work across the entire body. The pull-up is among the most basic exercise in calisthenics. While doing pull-ups you exercise your arms, your lower back muscles (especially those in the back, particularly lower) along with your abs and shoulders muscles, which work to keep your motor control in check and strengthening your whole body (especially the upper part of your body). Furthermore, as the muscles located in these areas are among of the most powerful, performing exercises that strengthen these muscles simultaneously results in a higher energy expenditure and, consequently, at the end of the day you will likely shed weight. This is not the only thing,

3: Leads to Weight Loss

When you exercise different muscles simultaneously it makes your body use the most energy (calories) This implies that by the time of the day, it is important to be aware of your diet--eat nutritious food and make a deficit of 500 calories a day, by the end of your week, you're likely to lose two weight or even more.

Most calisthenics workouts comprise compound workouts. Compound exercises require different muscles to work in harmony to increase particular movement patterns. For example, if you think about pull-ups you will notice that you employ your upper and lower body and arms to go through the movement. This, as you may expect, will ensure that your body is producing more energy in order to fuel the muscles.

Additionally while you are doing calisthenics workouts your lungs and your heart will be working harder to draw more oxygen to your body. This improves heart health, and when your breathing improves, also your capacity to deal with stress.

If you're putting on more fat, and you've tried everything you can --cardio or dieting, as well as weight training to shed the excess fat, calisthenics can prove extremely effective, as well as the benefits listed above, bodyweight exercises particularly when performed regularly can boost your metabolism. This means that Calisthenics the most effective method to shed extra fat.

4: Reduced Risk of Injury

When you stack the nature of a gym workout such as weighted squats against a calisthenics-adjacent exercise such as chaining a tire to your waist and pulling it, which of the two resembles a natural motion such as pulling game? It is evident that the former is the more natural. This is the appeal of calisthenics, where the exercises replicate the movements of nature. This is extremely beneficial.

In the beginning, if you've ever been to the gym more than a simple visit, then you are aware that among the numerous things that those who prefer exercise with weights complain about joint pains and problems. This is due to the fact that some exercises for weight training use joints in a completely unusual method.

When you do calisthenics exercise The movements and exercises are extremely natural. This means that you will experience a lower degree of injury as muscles perform well because the exercises are simple.

Furthermore, if you consider that the majority of weighted exercises focus on only one muscle, there is a chance that when you engage in weighted exercises in the gym it is possible to over-train specific muscles, leading to tears in your muscles. The fact that they don't focus on one muscle, can help prevent this. This helps improve the overall fitness of your body and, since you're working many muscles simultaneously which results in a well-sculpted body.

5: It's Not Monotonous

Although this book is not against weighted exercises, but if we're being honest While they're fun once you start however, after the initial enthusiasm wears down, the gym is a chore and exercising becomes monotonous particularly when you are forced to perform the same routine over and over again.

However the calisthenics are a source of creativity as with these exercises, there is an array of options to pick from. You can combine different exercises according to your preferences or increase your resistance anytime you'd like. Weighted exercises too have this feature, calisthenics provide an array of options that eliminate boredom from the scene.

6: Builds Lean Muscle Mass and Strength

If you're trying to build muscle mass then you should consider going to the gym and doing weighted exercises. But, there is some truth in the notion that calisthenics won't create a muscle-building body, if you're seeking a fit and robust body with a lot of well-sculpted muscles without needing to train with weights calisthenics is your most effective option.

Imagine a way to build chest muscles. There is a popular belief that in order to build strong chest muscles, you have to put on a ton of weight using your bench presses. Although this is true, the push-up is a classic yet effective exercise that will help you build massive lean chest muscles, especially in the event that you make your pushups more difficult through exercises like one-arm pushups, or even having your girlfriend lie behind you.

After having discussed the different ways that calisthenics will benefit you , and the reasons to take it up regardless of whether you're exercising You should be enthusiastic to start. The next part will go into exercises for calisthenics.

Chapter 2: Warming Up

Before you begin the most strenuous calisthenics exercises, beginning with warm-up exercises is recommended. Your goal is warming the most important body parts, like neck, calves and thighs, hips, shoulders back, arms, and shoulders. By doing this, your body is signaled to be ready for the coming sequence of intense activities. It will awaken your body. In delivering blood to those muscles you send the message that they'll be utilized during a long session.

Furthermore, the advantage of having warm-up exercises prior to major calisthenics exercise is the regulation of blood flow, enhanced range of motion, lower heart rate, and prevention. Since warming up allows you to engage your muscles throughout your body, you are less prone to pain in your back, joint pain, fractured bones, strains to soft tissue and muscle pains.

Four Simple Stretching Workouts

An exercise that is popular for warming up is stretching. In addition to benefits like controlled blood flow, increased range of motion, lower heart rate and injuries prevention, it's an effective method of mental conditioning. According to research that found it activates a portion of your brain to remain steady and calm regardless of any tension. Particularly when you're preparing for an intense workout of the specific type of weight training for the body It is best to train your mind not to allow yourself to be exhausted.

Four stretching exercises:

Stretching the buttock

Time:around 5 minutes

The specific benefit is that it strengthens the buttocks as well as nearby muscles

1. Relax on your back and lie down.

2. Bring both knees towards the chest.

3. Cross left leg across right thigh and then back to the left. Stay in this position for about 15 seconds.

4. Secure right thigh with a firm grip.

5. Right leg should be pulled towards chest.

6. Change the direction of crossover (between right and left legs).

7. Repeat five times with each leg.

Calf stretching

Time:around 5 minutes

Specific advantage/s:conditions calves

Instructions:1. By using the right leg, walk ahead.

2. Lean forward with a slightly straight right knee.

3. Maintain left leg straight while gradually lowering left leg.

4. With your heel set on the ground, keep in the same position for about 15 seconds.

5. Alternate between left and right legs.

6. Repeat 20 times on each leg.

Hamstring stretching

Time:around 5 minutes

Specific advantage/s:strengthens inner thigh

Instructions:1. Lay on your back and lift right leg.

2. With left foot placed on the floor, draw your left leg towards you; ensure that the right leg stays in straight place.

3. With both hands, grasp the inner thigh of the right leg. Stay in this position for about 15 minutes.

4. Repeat 20 times for each leg.

The inner thigh stretch

Time:around 10 minutes

Particular benefit/s: strengthens muscles in the the inner thigh, increases strength in the muscles in the thigh area

Instructions:1. Sit down, make sure your the back is straight.

2. Bend the legs and place your feet on the same side.

3. Keep feet in place, and gradually lowering knees towards the floor. Stay in

this the same position for approximately 15 seconds.

4. Do it 20 times.

Continuous Sessions

Regular calisthenics sessions can be exhausting, but, it is essential. When you are under the appropriate level of strain it increases your energy and your range of motion improved as you progress. Particularly, if you're thinking of an intense workout in the near future training yourself through the right exercises is recommended. According to the old saying, it's either you warm up or become swollen.

Three workouts per day:

1. Brisk Walk - Jumping Jacks - Huggers

Time:around 30 minutes

Particular benefit/s: slightly increases heart rate; increases the temperature of the shoulders, feet as well as chest, upper and lower back muscles as well as the lateral ones.

Instructions:1. Brisk walk for approximately 500 yards. Walk continuously for approximately 5 minutes.

2. Perform an exercise of jumping jacks (10 leaps).

2a. With your feet joined and your hands placed on either side, get up straight.

2b.Jump with your feet to the outside. Then, in totality, raise hands above head.

2c. Return to the starting position.

3. Complete the huggers in a series of (10 rounds).

3a. Straighten up.

3b. Move arms around the body.

3c. Abwehr arms until back is fully reached.

2. Jog - Arm Circles - Swingers

Time:around 30 minutes

Specific advantage/s:increases mental alertness; slightly elevates heart rate; warms up hips, legs, thighs, inner thighs, upper, mid, and lower back

Instructions:1. Jog lightly for 500 yards.

2. Do an arm circle (10 rounds).

2a. Straighten up.

2b. With your palms on the floor, stretch the arms out with both hands.

2c. Arms should be rotated in small circles.

3. Do an entire set of swingers (10 swings per leg).

3a. Get up straight.

3b. Move right leg backward and forward.

3c. Repeat with the left leg.

3. Run - Bent Huggers - Frog Jumps

Time:around 30 minutes

Particular advantage/s: slight increase in heart rate; helps warm up the legs, feet as well as chest, butt and the lower and mid back.

Instructions:1. Run for about 500 yards.

2. Do a set of bent huggers (10 intervals).

2a. Keep your knees bent.

2b. Wrap arms around the body.

2c. Repel arms until back achieved.

3. Perform Frog Jumps (10 jumping).

3a. Standing with feet separated Stand straight and upright.

3b. Set hands in the ground, then get into a squat.

3c. From the squat 3c. From the squat position, leap.

3d. Reach hands to head.

Chapter 3: Calisthenics Benefits And Constrains

CALISTHENICS BENEFITS

There's plenty to love about calisthenics, or bodyweight training. Calisthenics can refer to any exercise that you can do without using weights from HIIT to jumping jacks however, people typically refer to it as the strength training that is done with body weight for example, push-ups pushing-ups, and so on.

Let's look at some of the known benefits or advantages that take advantage of it.

Cheap or free.

There is no need for equipment to begin calisthenics. If you're just beginning in particular, you could complete a full workout on your flooring in your lounge.

(It might be beneficial to own a mat or Yoga mat but it's not essential at first.)

The beginning of the workout consists of basic movements, like:

Squats

Push-ups

Ab Work

All of them can be performed in the open air or on on a mat.

At first you will be able to exercise with no equipment. However, it is strongly advised to quickly begin adding push-ups or bodyweight lines to your workout routine.

If you don't perform these exercises, you'll not be able to exercise the back or biceps effectively. To do this, you'll require an adjustable pull bar (a basic one that's not fixed to the door) and/or a lower bar as well as parallel bars, a support for dip stands or something similar.

It gives you the chance of working out anywhere and at any time.

Calisthenics workouts are available and don't require much equipment, and you won't require much time or space for an effective bodyweight workout.

To get the best outcomes, you must take calisthenics as a routine workout program. Plan your time, keep track of your progress, and put in the full effort and intensity the workout program requires. (Don't only perform a few push-ups at times throughout the daytime.)

But, the exercises can be done in less than 30 mins at times, either outdoors or in the hotel room, on vacation or in the park at the table, anyplace you are able to stand up and lay down. Amazing!

A handful of exercise plans have this kind of ease.

*Weightlifting is a sport that requires special equipment that can be found in the gym or in a home gym . This will require a substantial sum of money for the setup to be in line with an established standard.

To stay fit and burn fats through running is a must. You need the use of a treadmill or spending some time outdoors and an environment that is safe for running.

If you're a busy traveler or want to make your life practical in all situations Bodyweight exercise with Calisthenics can help you in a greater way to achieve your ideal shape.

It's perfect for newbies because it's simple and is widely utilized.

If you're just starting to exercise, beginning with calisthenics exercises can teach you the right way to exercise safely before you can move on to weight training.

It incorporates full-body exercises, in contrast to traditional weight training and calisthenics routines are designed to bring the entire body in movement. This means that you can increase the strength of your entire body rather than focus on one area at one time.

It helps you move more easily in daily activities. Calisthenic exercises can be described as "functional" movements, which means they can help improve strength, coordination flexibility, stability, and coordination throughout your day, in addition to your gym or whatever exercise you choose to do.

Enhances flexibility, balance as well as mobility and stability.

Have you ever witnessed the bodybuilders or the strongmen who just cannot seem to get rid of their bodies clean?

This isn't the norm for bodyweight athletes who are extremely strong.

Maintaining your fitness through workout progressions will build immense strength and build a lot of muscle. It can also help you build remarkable strength and stability and also flexibility.

Advanced bodyweight exercises require a certain amount of flexibility to master, as well as strength and muscles.

If you're in search of an active and healthy body, then weight training could be the ideal option.

You are strengthened.

Calisthenics workouts help you increase your strength over time and make your entire body stronger with time.

In the end, calisthenics workouts are amusing.

Once you've mastered the fundamentals the calisthenics routine can help you to increase muscles and flexibility up to that you are able to do incredible things using your body that you were unable to accomplish before.

CALISTHENICS CONSTRAINS

Numerous advantages and plenty to admire the callisthenics exercises for However, some of the disadvantages might not be a good fit for a individual, especially those focused on a specific area or body part.

Physiotherapy

If you're experiencing an injury or undergone surgery, calisthenics may not be the most effective training for you. Following knee surgeries, it could be difficult to complete an squat with body weight. It is possible that you will require the assistance of an equipment.

The bodyweight exercises are essential however, you're performing too much work. Push-ups and push-ups are difficult if you're not strong enough. When you add a shoulder injury, the exercise will be impossible. Utilizing the use of a light dumbbell or a resistance band in your exercise routine, it can help you target specific muscle groups so that it becomes stronger and recovers. Calisthenics is a great exercise that uses lots of muscle, which leaves you with lesser control over injuries.

No exercise

Calisthenics can be extremely difficult, but you won't find the capability to travel for long distances, or to complete a lot of endurance exercises. Similar to weightlifting, bodyweight exercise is designed to help strengthen your. For best results you might want to include some cardio or aerobic exercises to increase your general fitness.

It might be a little difficult for newbies to begin.

Many newbies are disappointed or frustrated when they try to begin calisthenics, as the most "basic" movements are quite difficult for most people. The majority of beginners can do just a few push-ups. Many are unable to do even one push-up when they first start. This is how they could become bored and quit before they are ready.

Whatever fitness program you decide to follow, be sure to look for easy progressions that will assist you in getting started.

A progression is basically the process of changing your movement which help create more difficult moves. For instance, you can begin doing knee push-ups, or push-ups with band-assisted resistance until you're strong enough to be able to go forward.

Chapter 4: Calisthenics Routines For Beginners

In order to enhance your fitness, health and physique, it's essential to have an a routine that is effective to follow. Therefore, before we consider the best ways to climb to the highest point, let's familiarize ourselves with the fundamental calisthenics movements that you can begin practicing today.

Calisthenics, as we all know, is about making use of your body and weight to build muscle and build strength. This means that the majority of times, no equipment is required and you can complete many of these workouts with nothing except you and a amount of space.

More Difficult Calisthenics Exercises

In this article, we will speak about some of our popular exercises. You might already be familiar with some since they're well-known and you might had them in your practice.

Muscle-up

The muscle-up is one of the most popular exercise, but it is considered to be extremely difficult. Watching someone perform it flawlessly might make it appear easy however it requires lots of practice and endurance to be able to pull this movement down. Below are some steps you need to follow to take, and then try it and see if it is possible to do it!

Get a pull-up bar, then hold it by placing your thumbs on the top of it (this is a fake grip).

Now, you can pull yourself up. Your chin should be at that same plane as the bar.

Do a chest roll over the bars in order to switch into dips instead of pulling-up.

Finally, press your hands downwards to help you push your body upwards.

Experts agree that it's usually not the move that is difficult for people to master but gaining the strength to perform the move. Therefore, as you observe, this move will require many hours of training and practice. Therefore, you'll need to train to master this move.

Single Arm Handstand

The single-arm handstand isn't an easy one to master due to it being a task where you must to be steady and disciplined about your actions. However, with a bit of practice, it can be learned.

Then, starting from an upright position, place your palms on the ground , then move them off using your feet until you are able to keep your feet up in the air while your hands are supporting you weight.

Now, establish balance. Don't rush into lifting any of your hands off of the floor, instead do it slowly.

Take your hand slowly off the floor and let the weight of your body shift onto the hand still sitting on the ground.

Your legs must be a counterweight that helps keep you upright. If one of your legs is high to the other side, you may lose your balance and fall. Keep your core muscles engaged and keep your core engaged.

In order to master this technique it's important to ensure that you've mastered your balance and ensured you've got the strength to keep yourself upright long enough to keep the position.

Human Flag

The human flag is an sophisticated move can be mastered. It requires lots of strength in your legs, arms and core. It can be done on a ladder, pole or any other surface where you have an excellent grip. Here's how to perform it:

Start by choosing the appropriate pole. A sturdy, strong pole measuring around 2 inches in diameter could be the ideal one to begin however, remember that it's dependent on your personal preference. For those with larger hands, you might require a longer pole while people who have smaller hands may require smaller poles.

The most crucial aspect of this technique is the grip and the way you place your hands. It is recommended to put one hand underneath you for support, and the other hand over your head. Your palms must be placed in various places. Whatever you do with your hands, your body must be in the flag position, at a 90 degree angle after you've learned the technique.

Make sure your grip is secure to the pole be sure the arms remain aligned and that your arms are locked. Your legs should be swung into the air, and then lock them in place.

In this case, you'll need to move your legs around in order to achieve the 90-degree angle you want.

To get to this position, it may take many tries and will require lots of time to learn.

One Handed Planche

The one-handed planche is a highly advanced movethat is so complex that just a handful of individuals can master it all over the world. The exercise involves standing with one hand and keeping your body totally parallel to the ground. Here's how to perform the planche with one hand:

Begin on your knees.

Set both hands down in front of you , and then begin leaning forward on your hands.

When you are leaning forward, gradually move your legs forward and then dip your elbows into the abdominal area.

Slowly lift your legs out of the floor, until they're in line with your body and in line with the floor.

Then you'll be able slowly lift some of your fingers off of the ground. It is best to only take this the last time you're prepared and have reached a complete equilibrium.

The one-handed planche is intended as a holding device and not a dynamic movement. This means that motion is not required. Dynamic movement is the moment you move at all, even a little bit, while an hold is supposed to remain as steady as is possible.

Exercises for Absolute Beginners

We've learned a few of the more difficult moves are possible to master we can examine some moves you can begin learning now to build your way to the more challenging moves. These exercises are widely recognized, and you might already know how to perform them , and already have heard about them.

A few of these movements can be done at home, while some may require a amount of equipment such as an exercise bar with a pull-up feature or a wall pole of some kind However, these aren't difficult to locate or, in the event that you head to the gym, you will locate all of them there.

It is crucial to begin with a basic level when you're a beginner. This is because beginning at a level you aren't able to perform at could be dangerous for your health and the health of others around you, based on the workout you're doing.

Push ups

Push-ups can be beneficial when you want to build strength in your chest and arms. Before you can actually perform a push-up, be sure you are in the proper position. As you're lying on the floor, you should place your hands at shoulder width. Your feet should be placed in a place that's the most comfy for your body. This could be done by separating them or putting them joined. It is equally vital to ensure your body remains in a straight line.

Beginning in the correct shape for a push up Begin by bending your arms at the elbow and then tuck your elbows into the body.

Continue downwards to where your elbows sit 90-degree angle.

When your elbows are at 90 degrees, return to your starting position.

The push-up is a common movement and it's not uncommon that some people struggle performing it, especially if they're not particularly powerful. The practice, obviously can help.

Squats

Today, we've seen the squat, the workout which strengthens your legs and makes your body "pop." The squat gained popularity in 2015. However, it has been around for a long time. Everyone loves the feeling of a great leg workout and this is among the most effective ways you can build your legs.

Start standing in a position.

Begin to lean back like you are sitting in a chair, and bend to the knee.

Continue until your knees are parallel to your ground and you are knees at a 90 degree angle.

Keep your knees away from your toes, as that is poor posture and would not be as effective.

Pull-ups

If you've ever attempted pulling-ups at your local playground as young, you might have observed that it was quite difficult. Now you're large and strong and eager to do again, aren't you?

Begin by hanging from the bar using your hands held in a fake grasp (mentioned in the section on advanced moves).

With your arms and core, move your chin toward the bar.

When your chin is at the bar's level Once you have your chin level, you can let your body relax and move back to your starting position.

A few tips don't think of it as climbing up, but rather as you bring the bar towards your level. Many people view it this way and feel it makes the job seem easier.

Mountain Climbers

A mountain climber is designed to work the core and to burn calories fast by using your body weight. It is possible to do this workout easily by following these steps.

Put yourself in the pre-push-up position (straight back), with your legs in a comfortable posture and hands spread shoulder-width apart.

In this posture, bring your left knee towards your abdomen. Once your knee has been at the point that you are able to bring it then contract your abdominal muscles briefly but with force. This will assist in engaging the core.

After you have brought your left leg back into place, repeat the same thing using the right leg. Be sure to squeeze your abs whenever you bend your knee.

The reason this exercise is so efficient is because it's designed to be completed quickly. The rapid moving of your legs and tightening of abdominal muscles will make you feel a blaze fast.

Lunges

Lunges, similar to squats are intended to exercise your buttocks and legs.

Standing up Take a giant step forward using the left foot.

If you take your first big step ahead take your right knee and bend it until it's ready to touch the floor.

Just before your right knee is set to be on the floor, stretch your abdominal muscles, then bring the left knee back to the straight position from which you have been in since you started.

You can repeat it again using the other hand.

Walk Squats

A wall squat can be a form of exercise that targets the legs as well as glutes. Squats on the wall have been shown to boost the leg strength significantly like skiers do prior to their sessions in order in order to build their leg muscles prior to when they leave for the slopes. Here's how to accomplish it!

Sit on a wall with your feet spaced across your shoulders. Move off the wall (about two feet) with your back to the wall.

Then slide down the wall until that your legs are straight to the ground while your knees bend at an angle of a right angle.

Your knees should rest directly over your ankles. They should not go any more.

Continue this way for around 30 seconds, or as long as you're able.

Chapter 5: Warming Up And Increasing Mobility

It is important to warm up prior to any exercise, but more so when doing calisthenics. the intense contraction of muscles as well as just the sheer volume of muscles utilized in calisthenics make a solid warming up essential.

There are numerous situations where people take too much time warming up and slack off on bodyweight exercises. The result is disappointing results due to the fact that not enough time is put into the actual workout and exercises that are that are designed to build strength. Additionally the time spent in warm-ups could result in a lack of ability to do the exercises properly.

Warming up

The first step in the right warm-up has to do with good cardio, simply to increase your heart rate and make sure your muscles and tissues in shape. It is possible to start by jogging for a short time, since it is the simplest and does not require any equipment. Biking can be a fantastic method to get warm.

In essence, any activity that can get your heart rate going and your blood flowing and your muscles supple and warm will work. Be careful not to overdo it.

Flexibility and Mobility

Doing some stretching before doing calisthenics is essential since your ability to alter leverage also depends on your flexibility. Inability to get into specific positions can make it difficult to include resistance to your workouts.

Flexibility and stretching exercises don't only aid in your exercise, but they also help reduce knots, soreness, and tight spots throughout the body.

Flexibility can be divided into three primary components three main parts: lower body flexibility the core, as well as upper flexibility. While the importance of stretching is stressed in the media, as more flexible get the less you have to perform before exercise. It is easier to maintain flexibility rather than attain it.

*Note: There are certain stretch and flexes that require foam rollers.

Upper body

While upper body flexibility is usually neglected in favour of flexibility in the lower part of the body, since people are more likely to suffer from stiff hamstrings, it is nevertheless vital. Flexibility in the upper body is crucial when it comes to a successful performance when it comes to sports, and letting it go unnoticed will hinder your performance.

There are mobility and flexibility exercises for the entire shoulder. This includes the stretch-ups, pull-ups, as well as the dip of the scapula. Each one will be explained in detail.

Scapula Push-up

This strength and mobility exercise helps prepare you for the planche as well as the levers in the front and back.

Step 1: Place you in neutral position for a push-up.

Step 2: squeeze your scapula while stretching your chest toward the ground. Do not bend your elbows.

Step 3: When you've squeezed as hard as it is possible to squeeze, turn around the motions. Pull your scapula back and allow your spine and chest to lift. Your spine should be lifted as high as you can. Be sure not to turn your elbows.

Ten times repeat.

Pull-up of the scapula

This exercise will strengthen your shoulder muscles through your body's weight when you do this workout.

NOTE: You'll require a pull-up bars.

Step 1: Using the grip of your overhand hold the pull-up bar and hang it using your arms in a straight line.

Step 2: Lift your scapula. Shoulders should remain straight or even touching your ears.

Step 3: In this position of hanging, try to lower your scapula. Do not extend your elbows. Depending on the strength of your body you should be able to lift your chest. However, don't worry too much in the event that you're in a position that isn't possible. The strength will build as you continue the exercises.

Step 4: Hold your original position for a moment before returning to the position you started from.

Repeat 10 times.

Scapula Dip

This exercise builds the shoulders and helps you prepare for planches and handstands.

Step 1: Start in the triceps dip while maintaining your body's in a neutral position.

Step 2 Step 2: Lock your elbows and allow your body to sink down. Your shoulders should be raised and align with your ears.

Step 3: From this point move your body upwards while dropping your shoulders. At no moment during this exercise, move your shoulders.

Stretching the Chest and Shoulder

This next exercise is excellent for stretching the shoulders, armpits and chest.

Step 1 The first step is a floor workout. It is necessary to get on your knees and hands.

Step 2. While keeping your hips and buttocks aligned, move your body as near to the floor as you can. Make sure your arms are extended. Make sure to keep your shoulders and chest as close to the floor as you can to maximize the stretch.

Step 3: Keep the position for 20 minutes prior to release.

Torso

Since the core isn't as flexible as the lower or upper body parts, the exercise for strength and flexibility aren't as effective. The torso and spine don't provide much range of movements. However, this doesn't diminish the necessity of maintaining flexibility and mobility within the torso.

Spine foam rolls

This workout can reduce tightness and knots that are present in the muscles of the back and increase the ability of the spine to extend.

Step 1: Position the foam roller into a position which is at 90° from your body. The lower part of your back must be placed squarely over the roller while your feet are flat in the ground. Your hands should be at the ready to provide support when needed.

Step 2: Starting from the spine's base move back and forth across your foam roller. Make sure you slow down whenever you get into any sore places.

Third step: Keep to roll until you are at the top of your back. At this point, stop and attempt to make your spine rotate with the roller. This can open your chest and gives you greater flexibility.

Side Leans

Side leans can increase flexibility and mobility in the obliques, which is a very problematic area for many. In addition side leans also assist in increasing the mobility of the spine.

Note: You'll need the rod or bar for this exercise.

Step 1. Your feet should be spaced apart. Take the bar in your hands parallel to your feet. Then, hold the bar in front of your head. Your body should be in an X-shaped shape.

Step 2: Bend your body to one side in the waist, but without turning your back. Keep your arms as straight as possible. Make sure to keep the remainder part of you as straight as you can. Your waist is the only part of your body that is moving.

Repeat this 10 times.

Lower Body

Mountain Climbers' Exercise

This exercise is excellent to increase flexibility and mobility in the hips while at simultaneously stretching the hamstrings.

Step 1: Sit in the position that you will start from in the push-up. Your one leg must be raised in front of your hands while the other leg is spread out in front of you.

Second step: alternate your positions of your feet by making an elongated jump, then stretching the other side and moving the other foot to the side.

Do 10 times.

Frog Hops

This exercise is like climbing mountain climbers' exercises but with a bit more effort.

Step 1. Your starting position is the push-up position.

Step 2: Using an arc, move both feet forward with the right hand of your left hand while your left foot close to your left hand.

Step 3: After you've moved forward, jump backwards and return to the starting point.

Ten times repeat.

Knee Circles

This exercise significantly increases the mobility of the lower body. It opens up and opens the knees and hips.

Step 1: Take the position you started from. You must have your knees with your hands on the floor and your shoulder is aligned with your hands.

Step 2: Lift one leg towards the side while knee bent. Make sure the to lift it as high as is possible.

Step 3. With your knees bent, you can bring your foot forward until your knee is in contact with your arm.

Step 4: Once you have retreated from the previous position, return to your starting position , placing your knee back on the floor. You'll notice that your hips are making big circles using your hips.

Repeat backwards and forwards 10 times per side for both directions.

Chapter 6: Some Basic Calisthenics Exercises

In this section we will go over some of the most basic calisthenics routines. These techniques are designed to assist you achieve a more lean and more powerful body. Before beginning the exercises it is essential to understand the specifics of each and exactly how they should be done to get the most outcomes.

The exercises aim to strengthen your legs, arms and abdominal muscles. They also strengthen your oblique and more.

Warm-up exercises

All exercises in calisthenics must be preluded by warm up routines. Warm-ups assist in warming the body and preparing for the workouts. Make sure you do five minutes of warming up workouts to get your body ready for exercises in calisthenics.

Complete stretch

It is crucial to thoroughly stretch your body particularly your neck and back in order to warm up before the exercises.

Neck:

You can rotate your neck clockwise and anti-clockwise directions until you feel a slight stretch on the neck. Repeat this exercise for 10 repetitions.

* Now , move your head side-to-side so that you turn your head to the right and left. Repeat this 10 times.

* The final task involves bending your neck towards either side. Repeat this exercise 10 times.

For the back

The cobra pose is known to be among the best exercises for stretching your back and was adapted from yoga. To do this,

* Sit to the ground, with your stomach in contact with the ground.

Put your hands close to your chest, and then push your body up. Your lower torso must remain in contact with the ground while you raise your torso upwards.

Repeat this posture in 30 second increments each time, for five minutes.

The chest is for:

* Stretch your arms to either side.

Stretch your arms out towards the back, then bring them forward. Keep in mind to breath in and breathe out continuously throughout your workout.

Repeat the exercise ten times, while holding your hands behind for 10 seconds.

This will help you strengthen your chest. Make sure to breathe deeply.

For shoulders:

Exercise 1:

* Place your feet shoulder-length apart and hold your arms close to your sides.

* Now slowly move your shoulders, both in both directions.

Repeat the exercise ten times.

Exercise 2:

* Place your legs together and your arms at your sides.

Then, move your arms forward so that they're parallel to the ground. Begin to rotate your arms, but without bent them.

They should be turned clockwise 5 minutes , then making them counter-clockwise.

* Then you should bend your elbows, then place your shoulders on your fingers.

* Now turn your elbows clockwise as well as anti-clockwise movements.

Bend and stretch

The other kind of exercise is to stretching and bending. To do this,

Begin by bending your knees and rubbing your right foot using your left hand. Then, touch your the left foot using your left hand.

* Make sure to avoid bending your knees. If you have difficulty to begin it is possible to bend your knees a bit.

* Do this exercise continuously until you have 5 minutes.

Jumping Jacks

The most effective warm-up exercises is to do jumping Jacks. In actual fact, I'm sure many of you have done this workout before, in school or elsewhere. For this exercise,

Begin by standing with your feet close to each other and your arms by your sides.

Then, you leap up and raise your hands up and land with your feet separated.

* Jump back , then return to your original position. Repeat this until you reach the number of 50.

* Alternate these with the half-jumping jack with your hands instead of being raised up to the top, they're raised at a level parallel with the floor.

It is also possible to replace this exercise by an exercise called the Jumping Rope exercise if you have mastered the use of one.

Leg raises

For this warm-up exercise,

* Keep your legs in place and your hands by your sides.

* Straighten your right leg and then stretch your arms out.

* Try to place your left hand to your knee to the left.

* Lower your leg and repeat with the left leg.

• Repeat the exercise 10 repetitions for each leg.

If you've never done these exercises before, lay on a mat to practice this exercise. It is only necessary to feel your toes. When you're able be able to touch your toes then you are able to stand up and elevate your legs until they are in an ideal posture.

Twisters

Twisters are a simple exercise that can be done while sitting or standing up.

• Secure your fingers behind your neck and bring your elbows towards the front.

* Tilt your body to the left as far as your body can allow, then return in the same direction.

* Turn this to your left, then return it to the center. Repeat the exercise ten times.

Be aware of any back pains and be careful not to over-twist.

Arm and chest exercises

When you're done with the warm-up exercises, you can start to strengthen your arms and chest. Here are a few easy exercises to do.

Simple push ups

It is possible to begin your fitness routine with a few basic push-ups. To do this,

* Sit on your stomach and place your hands close to your chest.

Keep your feet in a straight line and point your feet to the floor. Balance your body.

* Now , raise your body using your hands until you are equal to the floor.

* Take a deep breath while in an upward position. Then exhale as you descend. Continue this for 3 to five minutes.

* When your body is getting stronger, you can do an additional variation of this workout. Instead of placing your fingers of the hand onto the ground you'll have to place your knuckles down on the floor.

Do push-ups for triceps

If you want to build your triceps, there's a particular exercise that will help you achieve it.

* Triceps can be found at the rear of your arms.

Place your palms on the floor with your index fingers and your thumbs should be in contact with one another to form an arc.

You should have your legs placed a bit away. Perform a push-up similar to any other push-up.

* Continue to maintain your breathing patterns before.

It may be a bit intense, but it's intended to increase the strength of your triceps.

Tricep Dips

If you are looking to strengthen your triceps muscles, there's a particular exercise to help you achieve it.

* Sit down on the bench and put your hands on the opposite the sides of your body.

* Now, shift your body to the edge of the bench.

• Lower your body until you are on the ground. Be aware that you don't need to get completely to the floor when you begin your exercise. Don't lean forward too much.

* Now, you can move your body up.

* Continue doing this for 15 times.

Push-up lifts

This exercise is designed to strengthen the chest muscle. This is why,

Set the legs of your feet on an elevated platform , such as a chair or sofa.

Continue to push-up as a normal push up.

Plank to Push Up

This workout strengthens your shoulders, arms and your core.

Begin by bringing your entire body to the plank in a straight line.

Put your hands on the mat, shoulder length. Then, lift your body up.

* Bring your legs towards the back.

* Lower your body as if you were doing a push-up and then return to your plan posture.

Exercises for the abdomen

Many suffer from abdominal fat that can be difficult to shed. Here are a few easy exercises you can do to strengthen the abdominal muscles.

Lower abdomen exercises

Simple Crunch

It is a very well-known exercise that could hurt your back if you don't do it correctly.

* Lay on the floor and put your arms by your side.

* Bend your knees , bend them and lift your feet off the floor.

Keep the height at 6 inches above the ground. Your legs from knee to the feet must be straight to the floor.

Then, bring your knees to your chest, and then try to reach them.

* Your upper torso needs to be secured to the floor whenever you are doing this.

Perform three sets, with the same number of repetitions for each set.

Cross crunch

This is a fantastic exercise to build the ablique muscles. To do this exercise,

* Sit in a position on your floor. Then, lift your legs and bend your knees.

* Cross your right leg over your left leg. Your foot that is resting must be on the opposite knee.

* Lift your upper body off the floor till your elbow is in contact with your left knee. Repeat on the opposite side.

* Return to the original position.

Repeat this process till you can feel the burning in your lower abdomen.

Cross stretch

To do this exercise,

* Lay to the ground and bend your knees as you would for a basic crunch.

* Now, extend your left hand towards the right leg. Repeat the opposite side.

* Keep switching. Do between 15 and 20 repetitions.

Plank Progression

This workout will strengthen your calves and your core. You'll need to move gradually from the initial plank position, to the final position of plank.

* Place your body on your back. Set your forearms firmly onto the mat.

• Lift the body upwards and keep the core muscles tightly. You can also squeeze your butt muscles.

* Hold this position for 30 seconds. Gradually increase the amount of seconds.

Once you feel at ease with this posture You can then begin to perform this exercise while your arms are extended onto the mat.

* To take it another step forward, put your legs on a platform inclined and then perform the exercise.

It can be done in the opposite direction. It is necessary to lay on one side for this exercise. Similar steps are applicable for this one too.

Exercise for the legs and butt

Here are some easy exercises to strengthen your legs.

Simple kicks

* Sit down on the ground with both your hands resting on the floor and your knees firmly on the floor. You'll appear like an animal.

Begin to gently move your right leg inward until it is straight so that your leg is at an angle of 45 degrees. Keep in mind that your knee shouldn't reach the floor.

* Repeat this 10-12 times, and then switch legs.

Be careful not to do it too quickly as it can cause injuries.

Basic Squats

To do these squats

* Place your legs set slightly apart.

* Stand up with arms raised so that they are in line with the ground.

Then, slowly sit down in a squat posture. Keep in mind that your knees should not be bent, and your arms should be at a level with the floor.

Slowly raise to return to the original position. This is the end of one repetition.

* Repeat the exercise 25 times.

Squat jumps

Squat jumps are easy and efficient exercises to strengthen your legs. It is possible to invest a bit of effort in order to complete these.

* Place your feet in the same squat position , then do a squat.

Jump up instead of falling and return back to the position of squatting. This is a single repetition.

* Repeat the exercise 25 times.

Glute Bridges

This exercise targets your glutes as well as your hamstrings.

* Sit in a reclined position on the back. Your arms can be stretched out to either side of your lower body in a 90-degree angle with respect to your body. Bend your knees.

Now, take an inhale and then lift your hips up to the ceiling and exhale. Keep this posture for 10 seconds. Be sure to engage your core muscles as well as those in your butt muscle.

* Take another breath , then exhale as you bring you back on the mat.

* Repeat this exercise 10 times.

Lunges

This workout is extremely beneficial to strengthen your butt muscles and legs. There are three different variations of this exercise: front lunges, the side lunges and back lunges. Let's take a glance at front lunges. The two other variations are basic variations that this one.

* Place your mat on the floor with your feet shoulder-width away.

* Put your hands across your chest.

Now, bring your right leg toward the front while keeping the knee bent. Be sure that your foot remains straight. The left leg needs to be stretched with your foot in a straight position. Maintain this position until you notice a stretch in the left of your leg. Your back must be straight all the time.

* Return the right leg towards the center and do the same exercise for the other leg. This creates one set.

* Repeat the sequence 10 times.

* For side lunges, it is important to have to shift your leg towards the side and then back to do back lunges.

Chapter 7: A Tale Of Caution

Things to watch out for are:

Remember that your primary and most priority is you health as well as the condition of your physique. It is not worth getting to the top of Calisthenics when your body is likely to get weakened and you will not reap the rewards of your efforts. Therefore, don't exercise so much that you overwork yourself, a situation known as "training to failure" where your exercise routine could cause irreparable injuries to your muscles and bones due to being too enthusiastic, or confused. Never quit ignoring the discomfort in your tendon because of rupture that could cause you to require surgery to repair it and be in a position to move your limb in the same manner ever again. While it might sound terrifying however, it's also highly unlikely. It is essential to be aware that even though your body is an imposing beast of a machine, capable of lifting double its weight in order to keep the same level of efficiency,, your body requires adequate time off and proper nutrition. All of it must be maintained within a reasonable amount, just as the food you eat and the amount you spend. If you consume too much food, you'll become overweight and If you spend too much on things that you do not want, you'll find yourself financially strained at the end the month. It doesn't mean that eating out or shopping bad but it means that you must find an option to balance how much you'll spend and the amount you need to put aside.

Medical complications that could be a concern:

Form of Bad:

Training should be performed at a precise angle, because you'll be bent and being pushed against the forces of gravity. There are areas which are dependent and have to perform more than other parts to hold the weight of your body, specifically your back. This is the reason why you find trainers focused on keeping their clients' backs straight or giving additional support for the back. The back of your body is home to some of the most powerful muscles you have, however they are prone to strain. If you begin to feel that your back is becoming too fatigued or begins to ache, particularly in the region of your lumbar (that is the area in your lower back which naturally curvatures) you should take some time and consult an instructor or trainer to help you improve your posture. The the correct posture and posture for each exercise in the next section.

Strains: Spraining ligaments is not unusual in the world of sports, it's the result of stretching or twisting of ligaments which causes inflammation, however it is not dislocation. Sprains take healing time, however the majority of joints require some degree of mobility, even if injured. This will prevent the joints from stiffening following recuperation. If you suffer from sprains, consult your physician. In the event of an emergency, the best option for emergencies is the RICE rule rest, ice compression and elevation. take the time that is needed Do not immediately jump into the same level of exercise and allow your body the time to heal. The application of ice to inflamed areas aids in the healing process, and also reduces the pain. Bandages that are compressed provide the limb support, and reduces discomfort. The elevation, especially in the lower limbs, helps prevent blood pooling and inflammatory mediators from building up within the injured areas, making the healing process speedier.

Extra Strain to the muscle:

A certain amount of stress is necessary in order to build muscle and enhance strength, but this should be done gradually It is not recommended to go for a long time committing yourself to many hours of exercising without breaks to see quicker results. The over-use of your muscles may cause fatigue after a workout that can affect your workout schedule the next day, only creating more stress, which can make you exhausted throughout the day, triggering the cycle of fatigue.

Excessive muscle contraction can result in a condition referred to as Rhambdomyolysis. Excessive muscle contraction can cause microscopic tears and break down of the muscle, leading to blood in the urine and painful pain at the muscles's site of injury. It may also result in muscles tear and tears in the tendon.

These issues are easily avoided by giving yourself plenty of relax. If you are feeling that pain isn't a typical discomfort due to being in a high-flying position or you experience a sensation that is unusually high enough that getting started hurts, slow off the speed of your workout and do not exercise at the maximum intensities. While the ailments aren't common, they could be fatal, so it is essential to exercise precautions. Regular exercise is a great way to stop most of these issues. You don't want to put in the effort to achieve your goals and then end up in bed and then lose the gains you've made. There are no shortcuts to getting well; it was years of a poor lifestyle to achieve the body you are today, therefore, be patient with yourself because it may take some time for your body to behave exactly how you want it to be. You are your body's best resource, so make the most of it.

No play and all work

Be sure to take pleasure in your workout. Calisthenics is challenging , and If you're someone who enjoys taking on the challenge, you'll be entertained by the way your body is progressing , however even the most interesting Calisthenics routines can get boring as time passes. It is essential to be happy with whatever you're doing. This helps keep you focused and remain dedicated to your goal. There are plenty of exciting activities that you can engage in to work out in a different way every now and again, all you need to do can you switch up your routine to can help you tone and shed fat. Everything from low-cardio like rock climbing and hiking to high-intensity biking swimming, or even try an activity with a group! Whatever you can do is something you should consider trying. So you won't skip out on the daily tasks you carry out.

If you are bored and do not exercise on one day, you're likely to skip out in the future and you'll lose interest in training, particularly in the beginning of your training.

It's vital to have fun working out This will help you get those. It is possible that you don't like working out to work out. It is possible that you need to incorporate a bit more variety to your exercise routine. Whatever the reason, there are plenty of activities that will can tone your muscles and burn fat.

Get a friend together! Create a group of people who would want to train together. If you're a student at university or working at a place of employment, post a notice on the wall inviting people to become your workout partner. The people who join in add entertainment and some level of competition, which makes exercise more enjoyable. Working out in a group with could also offer different workout venues. Training in the same spot for a prolonged time frame can cause the entire experience to become dull. While it's important to stay to a particular spot to establish the habit A change in setting can be beneficial in making your workouts more enjoyable.

Chapter 8: A Snapshot Of Mental Success

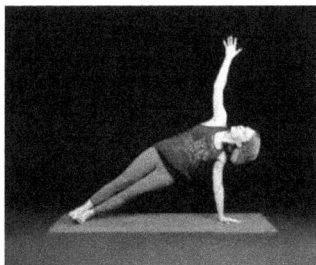

In this segment, we'll examine how having a powerful and positive mental picture of ourselves is essential for us succeed with calisthenics. If you envision you are doing these exercises throughout your life positive affirmations will be more easy to attain.

Your mind ought to be filled with positive images of health, energy and feeling healthy. Image boards and other tools can aid in forming a complete mental picture.

This List Matters:

* Image boards must be clear on the goals.

Learn to handle the problem of cravings and lack of motivation.

* Properly constructed imagery to increase motivation and self-esteem.

Positive body image and how holding that image inside your head influences your subconscious to alter the body's shape.

Keeping A Vision Board:

Vision boards don't need to be expensive and is simple to make. A cardboard piece with a couple of color markers are all that you require, particularly if do not have access to lots of money.

Find photos of poses that stretch or capture screenshots of calisthenics exercises and post them onto your board of vision. Indicate how many repetitions and how often you'll be doing this exercise. You can rate the exercise between 1 and 10 as simple or difficult for you to complete. Continue to choose other images from the internet until you are able to figure your entire program out.

Place the vision board in a prominent location in a place where you can you can see it.

Everyone has things they do not like, such as squats, push-ups, or push-ups however, the vision board suggests that you must get healthier and fitter, then these workouts are essential. The ability of a strong brain can help push us past these mental obstacles and provide us with a feeling of satisfaction when done.

How to deal with cravings Do you currently have a photo of yourself that makes you feel sad? That's the one that makes you cringe whenever someone sees it. When you have a photo that is unattractive can help you curb your cravings as when you are feeling like cheating using the sexy image will allow you to keep your stance.

A trick to help with Hunger: Fill an oversized glass with water and squeeze 2 tablespoons of lime or lemon juice into the cup, add two tablespoons Apple Cider Vinegar and drink it down. Both of these combinations can aid in reducing the appetite and hunger, increase metabolism, reduce blood sugar levels and help improve digestion.

Concerning Body Image: A lot of women are unhappy with their body because that they must look in a certain way, but it's not a realistic image of females.

Restoring your body and mind can also mean creating a realistic picture of the person you are as a person, which includes the body shape. The most commonly used female body types are Apple, Banana, Pear and Hourglass that define their size, metabolism and weight. It is possible to calculate your body type by clicking the link below to find the figure for your body's type.

Source:

https://www.calculator.net/body-type-calculator.html

Our bodies are of all forms and, while everyone can alter their body shape There are certain genetic traits passed down from your parents that are unchangeable.

Depending on whether you're curvy or straight, these exercises can help you shape your body and target the problem areas.

This is the time to determine the most effective calisthenics for your body type to increase your shaping. Learn more about it later. ....

There's no reason to think we can't modify our calisthenics routines in order to fit better into our body's shape. Don't be afraid to try various exercises to are a good fit with calisthenics. In the end, the objective is to build an athletic, healthy and flexible body.

Psychological Hacks To Maximize Physical

Growth

As with everything else we be tempted to attempt in our lives There will always be an learning curve that goes along with it. Exercise is no exception and every person has strengths and weaknesses that we must overcome.

Understanding the rhythms and capabilities of our bodies can take some time and we need a bit of motivation to get through the dark days. It's fine to enjoy couch potato at times but you must never forget what you want to achieve. There's no problem with having one or two days off from working out. The back slide and loss of motivation that you must be aware of.

One way to stay out of this depression is to become your own counselor or therapy therapist. Keep a written document of precisely what you're doing.

Note down your daily eating habits, workout routine, and emotions each day, will aid in your progress and will keep your mind healthy.

About Psychological Hacks These hacks target and target areas of concern we have to address. Hacks prevent us from consuming high-fat, sugary food items, feeling lazy and exhausted, or losing hope in the face of frustration. Hacks are tiny messages sent to the brain that keep us in the loop.

Imagine having your very own personal coach on your shoulder and whispering "Keep going, just look at how amazing your body is starting to look!" A customized hack program can boost your motivation levels physically as well as emotionally.

Here are some motivational strategies I would like you to employ daily:

Positive Reinforcement is an extremely beneficial way to exercise when you're getting fit because there will be occasions that you'll be exhausted and stiff. Positive reinforcement can help guarantee that you'll continue to push even when you don't desire to.

Write down a record of all your activities You will find very solid psychological reasons for me to suggest the same practice. It can train your brain to change from 'I think I'm capable''I'm sure I can'. In time, you'll be able to revisit to see how you've progressed and perhaps assist someone else who may also require some encouragement.

* How to reinforce good Conduct: Who says you can't be rewarded for all the effort? Rewarding good behaviour can include buying a brand new item of clothing or enjoying an ice cream treat every week.

Even if you work five days a week, doesn't mean you shouldn't indulge yourself in some time. If children are doing something right and behave well, their parents would like to acknowledge their good behavior with a sweet reward. But guess what? the similar rules will apply to your work too!

If we exercise regularly and stick to our program by rewarding yourself with a special reward can be a positive way of preparing for long-term achievement!

Shaping using intermittent reward-based (R+) is a tool to overcome mental blocks and plateaus. This could occur when we reach the point in our exercise program where our body does not appear to be moving forward. When this happens , individuals will occasionally feel the need to give up or putting off Calisthenics.

Everybody experiences a plateau, however, be aware that this too will come to an end. After you've lost some weight or have toned the body up to some level it is possible to come to an time when you'll reach a point where you are at a level.

Another thing I think should be addressed when you're not altering your diet and increasing your intake of calories generally, this is the time when people reach an unsustainable level. The body needs more energy to build muscle mass, and if it isn't getting this, it will eventually are more frequent. The physical signs you might observe when you reach an unsustainable level are as follows:

It feels like you're losing your strength.

Feeling flushed more than usual.

You may have noticed a decline of your appetite.

* Feeling like giving up and feeling uneasy.

* Heart rate changes during rest cycles.

Feeling tired, with less motivation.

* Irritable , with unproven aggression.

* There is no new growth in the mass of muscle (10 -14 days).

* If you aren't feeling motivated, avoid any workout that requires weights and body lifting.

Typically, plateaus last a few weeks before your body will begin to transform muscles from fat So, stay focused and you'll get through this stage of your evolution.

Utilizing "Self Speak" like a super-coach to help you reach the next step: I'm sure you've heard about affirmations and messages to the heart? Self-talk is all about positive affirmations that you affirm your self-talk every day. Maintaining peace and happiness through any exercise routine is very beneficial to the body and mind.

Self-talk can be about finding positive words from people who have accomplished their goals and can inspire you. Find mentors who can have a positive influence on your mood and mental health, will allow you to keep you in a positive state. If you are suffering from depression, self-talk is essential, particularly when we are feeling depressed or are unable to accept negative thoughts about our lives.

*4 corner/military training to overcome obstacles Doctor. Thomas L. DeLorme was an Army doctor who realized the need to assist those returning from War in 1948. They needed physical rehabilitation and strength training. Many were weak because of the harsh living conditions and the absence of food items that were fresh.

DeLorme developed a program that was based on numerous set of repetitions which is 10 repetitions being the highest for every exercise that the patient completed. If the patient did pull-ups, he'd do 4 set of 10 reps.

The program was later referred to as "Progressive Resistance Exercise," which gyms all over the globe still practice in the present. If you hire an exercise instructor, they would suggest repetitions for every exercise they want you to complete.

In the next chapter of the book, we'll be taking a look at Calisthenics and their benefits for people who wish to understand more about the history behind them.

Chapter 9: What Is Bodyweight Training?

Prior to the invention of equipment and machines for exercise, people who wanted to build strength and muscle were required to work out using their body weight. While this idea was initially developed because there was no alternative, it's a method of exercise that is still utilized in the present due to its effectiveness.

The practice of bodyweight training has a long-standing history and has been a regular component used by military groups for many years. This is most likely due to the fact that bodyweight training being relatively inexpensive, and also the ease that it does not require any special equipment, and thus it can be performed almost anywhere.

In addition to the military applications the bodyweight exercise continues to be utilized in the world of athletics and also play an important element in the majority weight loss and muscle growth exercises that are available across the world.

When we take a look at an entire program that incorporates weights, also the bodyweight exercise has particular advantages and benefits, with the bodyweight exercise has been proved to be efficient in general exercise that is bodyweight-based are vastly different from most weight-bearing exercises, even if similar muscles and exercises are utilized.

Why are they distinct?

Bodyweight exercises like lunges, push-ups as well as other exercises belong to a category of exercises referred to as close Kinetic Chain Exercises. These are the exercises in which the foot or hand is fixed and doesn't move independently of the surrounding body.

If these exercises are compared to other exercises like leg curls, bench presses and leg curls, they are part of the group of movements known as open chains of kinetics. They are executed without the foot or hand being fixed, and allows movement in conjunction with the rest of the body.

If the body moves in the direction of or away from an object , the chain is closed. However, if you move anything away or towards from your body is open.

There's a vast distinction between someone pulling themselves toward an object , and pulling an object toward them when they are in a fixed posture with regards to both neuromuscular and muscular stimulation. The addition of closing kinetic chains using bodyweight into your training program stimulates your neurological system in different manner than open exercises in kinetic chain. There are closed chain kinetic exercises that are thought to be superior because they require many muscle groups to work together when moving.

Combining open and closed Kinetic chain exercises

While open chain kinetics exercises may be more effective than bodybuilding exercises or strength training that combines both will always be able provide you with the most effective results.

Combining various exercises exposes the brain to various types of stimulation and increases the efficiency , therefore a combination between CKC exercise and OKC exercises can help boost your strength as well as the tone.

It is also important to note that because there is no equipment required, it is easy to move from one activity to the next with ease, that not only saves time, but an effective way to keep your time off shorter, your heart rate high and increase the speed of your metabolic rate.

Training with bodyweights isn't just beneficial on its own but when it is incorporated into an exercise routine that incorporates weights, it can also increase the effectiveness of.

The bodyweight exercise is the perfect option for anyone of all ages and degree of fitness.

Chapter 10: Back & Abs

A bent-over Dumbbell rows. 3 sets with 10-12 repetitions. 30-40 second rest in between sets.

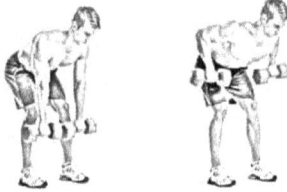

Execution Stand at a shoulder width apart with feet with your knees bent slightly take 2 dumbbells using the grip of your overhand. Then, lean forward with you hips, until the waist is aligned to the floor. The dumbbells should be straight in front of your shins. With your body not raised and pulling the dumbbells upwards, you should pull them up toward your abdomen, keeping your elbows up and above your back's level. The dumbbells should be held in the position of peak-contracted for a short time before slowly lowering them down the same route.

Pull-ups in doorway (Doorway pullup bar) 3 sets 10-12 repetitions. 30-40 second rest in between sets.

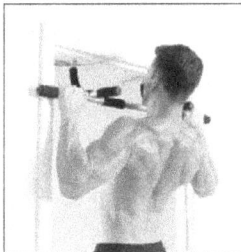

Execution - Grab an overhead bar and use a broad overhand grip, and wrap your fingers across the bar. You can choose between a tight and broad grip of your discretion. Lean back with ease from the bar with arms extended fully and your legs crossed behind your. Engage your lats to lift your body up, focusing to keep your arms toward your sides and lifting them towards your back to lift your own body. Pause for a moment as your chin is raised or crosses the bar's level and then lower yourself without locking at the lower end. Keep your elbows slightly tucked in throughout the exercise, without movement that is jerking or swinging. It is possible to purchase the bars from a local sports products shop.

ABS - Planks

3 sets, however many you are able to reps. 30-40 seconds rest between sets.

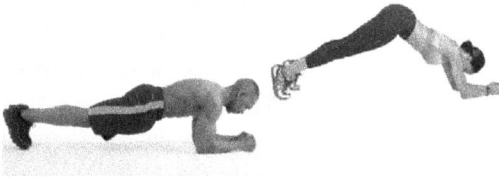

Execution: Begin by lying on mat. Put your forearms onto the mat, with your shoulders aligned with your elbows. Place your hands on top of your. Spread your legs behind you and then rest your feet on your toes in a similar way to if you were doing pushups. Your hips shouldn't be elevated to the ceiling or the back of your body be arched. It is important to aim for a straight lines between your toes and shoulders.

The abdominal muscles should be tightened to ensure you can hold the correct position and keep it the longest you can. If you notice your lower back begin to feel tired then take a break and then return to the proper posture and repeat the exercise again. Keep your breathing evenly throughout the movement. It's a common mistake to try to keep your breath in the exercise however, it'll be more effective if you concentrate on breathing in a uniform manner. By doing this, you'll be able to supply oxygen into your muscle, and makes to keep them strong for longer. Sometimes, I'll even move my hips upwards and downwards with a controlled, slow motion. (as if you were being sexually active lol)

You can feel your abdominal muscles becoming fatigued and working when you hold the position. Make it a goal to hold the posture a bit longer each time you exercise. Try to hold the position for 30-60 seconds the first time. If you experience pain on your lower back, you're performing the exercise incorrectly, and you are likely to let your back sink. Keep a straight and stable lower back throughout the your exercise.

Chapter 11: Ways To Get Fit, Lose

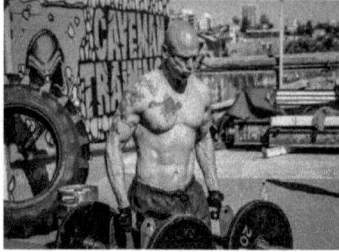

Weight, And Feel Better

Building up the Right Mindset

Create the right attitude. The psyche might not be a muscle, however it's still incredibly solid and has the ability to make a difference between succeeding but not achieving your goals. Fitness is a long-distance race and not a walk that requires changes to your entire way of life. Do not give up in the event that you don't get what you're looking for.

Don't approach this with the idea that you will stop the progress you've made once you've reached your goal of fitness at a high level or else you could fall into your old habit again. Fitness should be about integrating aspects of your life that you can eventually accomplish through habit.

Be aware of your progress and enjoy minor improvements.

It's a good idea to create a "fit journal to ensure to track your progress while working out, the activities you engage in and how much you exercise. It is also possible to record the food you consume each day. It is possible that if you are required to note whether you have nibbled or not, you are less likely to eat.

Don't think that there is a reason why, if you face a particular issue that you have to abandon the entire thing and give up to the world. Don't be discouraged even if you have stopped losing weight or building muscle mass; remember that plateaus are not uncommon, however overall , you are on the upward path and that's definitely something to be proud of.

Sign a commitment contract with yourself.

They are also referred to as an incentive system. Create a goal for yourself, and then decide on a reward that you will be able to enjoy. Choose something you'd like to do or one that you'd like to do.

To celebrate set a goal with you that if you can run for 30 minutes continuously then you will be able to buy the perfect shirt or golf clubs you've thought about over the last few weeks.

Find a friend to comfortable together.

It's much easier to accomplish your goals when there is an individual to share the burden and success with. Create a plan that you can both concentrate on and keep on the right track.

You can even bring an entire group of people on the "get fit" program. Everyone should put $10 in an account, and the one who works out the most during the time period that is speculated wins the money.

Exercising to Get Fit

Include exercise in your daily schedule.

Set the alarm, get up, eat at the table, get your children for school, and then work for about 8 to 9 hours. get the kids up from school, cook dinner after soccer training after which shower and clean the house... Exercise? Maybe tomorrow sounds like a routine? Do you believe that you are among many people trying to figure out a suitable place to fitness?

It's a common misconception that in order to achieve the best exercise , you need to work approximately an hour in the gym.

More and more, research suggests that there's a significant benefit in incorporating brief episodes of exercise into your routine activities. And without visiting the fitness center! According to an ongoing report from the American Council of Exercise, brief periods of exercise lasting less than 10 minutes are beneficial to lose weight. Additionally, NHANES examine the more breaks the members took, the slimmer their waistlines and the less C-responsive protein levels they had (a measure that indicates inflammation). It is also clear that, without question, a breaking from an inactive lifestyle can help blood sugar levels. Every minute of exercise is important. Feel content knowing that the stairs instead than the lift, and picking the most pristine parking spot at the entrance aren't wasteful!

Simple ways to incorporate an exercise routine into your day:

Do you work at a desk? You should keep a water bottle near the desk area. You can fill it up halfway, in the hope to fill it close to refills throughout the day.

If we'd prefer not to make it publicly known or not, television typically consumes an hour or so in our daily lives. In every break in the office take 20 triceps seat dips and feel the heat. In the opposite direction you can turn off the evening's television show and go for a stroll or bicycle ride.

At the end of each hour, make sure you roll your chair into the opposite direction to your workplace and do squats for 20 seconds. Followed by ten full squats.

repeating. Set an alarm on your phone for you to be reminded of your obligation to rise every hour!

Schedule buddy system! Make a conscious effort to plan two or three "breaks" in your day with a coworker and attempt an exercise circuit. It'll only take two minutes!

On your forearms hold an ordinary plank during 40 seconds.

Turn your body over onto your left arm to do a side plank and hold it for 40 seconds.

Turn your left arm to complete the final side plank and hold for 40 seconds.

If you are thinking about the possibility that the water may bubble, or the stove is pre-warming take your time doing bent push-ups at the counter.

Are you able to find a major webinar or conference call you can join this morning?

Have your dumbbells handy! Smash in bicep twists extension of the tricep and shoulder presses during the commotion. You won't be able to tell!

Do you have a baby who is fighting naptime? Do side lunges to "rock" your infant to take a nap.

In your yard, try to bend and pick dandelions and other weeds that you don't want. This will provide three benefits exercising, beautiful garden and no need to apply harmful herbicides.

The interval between school plays or during the half-time of any sporting event is a great moment to go for a 5-10 minute energy walk in the corridors or around the school while you're supporting your children.

Plan effective date evenings! If it's time spent with your loved child or with your partner Avoid dinner and film and go for something active! Cook your meal at home, walk to the most beloved park or bike around the area or perhaps play tennis... or take an PFC picnic lunch and find an amazing spot to take in the view!

Are you unable to find the time to go through an hour of a workout or a personal training session? Don't be too stressed about it. These ten methods to make your body move be beneficial! If you are in a position where your body requires reaching to push, pull and pivot, squat, or squat... Include some repetitions! Every movement counts, therefore you should make the most of it.

Exercise and eating

Eat a balanced breakfast

If you're planning to work out during the early morning hours, get up early to eat breakfast not less than an hour prior to your workout. You should be well-fueled prior to starting the gym. Research has shown that drinking sugar or eating it prior to exercise may improve the efficiency of your workout and allow you to exercise for longer periods or greater energy. If you don't consume food, you might feel lightheaded or sluggish while exercising.

If you plan to exercise within an hour following breakfast, you should have an easy breakfast or consume anything, e.g., a sports drink. Emphasize carbohydrate for greatest energy.

Breakfast options that are great include:

Whole-grain oats , bread or whole grain oats

Low-fat drain

Juice

A banana

Yogurt

Hotcakes

Be aware that If you typically drink espresso in the mornings, drinking a container prior to your workout is probably fine. Remember that if you try eating or drinking in the first place prior to exercising, you run the risk of building developing a bitter stomach.

Size is everything

Be aware; don't push to be too strict when it comes to the amount of you consume your food prior to exercising. The general guidelines suggest:

Big meals: eat this between three and four hours prior to working out.

Small snacks or meals Eat this for between one and three hours before exercising.

In excess food intake prior to exercising can make you feel tired. If you eat too little, it won't provide you with the energy needed to keep in good shape during your exercise.

Snack well

The majority of people can have small portions of food prior to or during their workout. It's all about what you're feeling. Find what is most comfortable for you. Consuming snacks prior to exercise likely won't give you more energy if your exercise is less than an hour long, however, it could help curb hunger cravings. If your workout lasts longer than one hour, you could benefit by having a carbohydrate-rich meal or drink to fuel your exercise. The best snacks include:

A bar of energy

Apple, a banana or other fresh fruit

Yogurt

Fruit smoothie

A whole grain bagel or wafers

A granola bar with a low fat content

Peanut butter sandwich

A sports drink or dilute juice

A nutritious snack is crucial if you're planning to do to exercise for a couple of hours following a meal.

Eat after you exercise

In order to allow your muscles to heal and replenish glycogen stores, consume food that is rich in protein and carbohydrates in the two hours following your workout session, if you can. The best post-workout meals include:

Natural fresh fruit and yogurt

Peanut butter sandwich

Chocolate drain with low-fat and pretzels

Smoothies to help you recover from your workout

Turkey is served on bread made of whole grains, with vegetables

Drink up

Make sure to drink plenty of fluids. You should drink enough fluids prior to or after exercising to avoid dehydration.

To stay hydrated during exercising to stay hydrated, the American College of Sports Medicine recommends that you:

Drink between 2 and three cup (473 or 710 milliliters) of water just a few hours prior to your exercise.

Drink about 1/2 to one Cup (118 up to 237 milliliters) of water every 15-20 minutes throughout your exercise. The amount you drink should be adjusted according to your body's size and conditions.

Drink between 2 and three cup (473 up to 710 milliliters) of water following your workout for every one pound (0.5 kg) of weight loss in the course of your workout.

Water is typically the most effective way to replenish lost fluids. However, if you're training for more than an hour you should drink a sports beverage. These drinks can help keep your body's electrolyte balance and boost your energy since they're loaded with carbohydrates.

Chapter 12: Calisthenics Equipment For Competent Workout

Calisthenics workouts are known for their simplicity, making it possible to be done without the use of any equipment. This chapter could be contradictory to the first statement, but I believe it's essential to consider some of the equipment that can help aid in your workouts. For instance, it's simpler to get an exercise bar that you can pull up for your pull ups , rather than searching for different items to use around the home. What are the tools you require for effective calisthenics exercise?

(i) Then pull up the bars

Like the name implies, they are utilized to perform pull-ups. It is the first thing to buy one of these machines, preferring one with the longest distance from the wall due to the movements. Then, go to your home and mount it on your wall. It's as simple as it gets.

(ii)Gymnastic rings

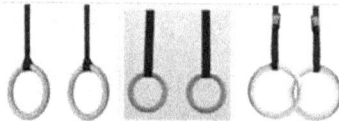

A gymnastic ring gives the possibility of taking your bodyweight exercises to the highest level. In the beginning, rings work various muscle groups within your body. It requires lots of energy to maintain balance, so it coordinates all of your body parts, which gives you a full exercise.

(iii) Abs wheel

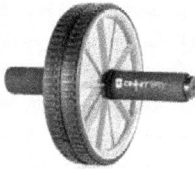

This machine is mostly employed to help strengthen your abdominal region i.e. abs. What is its purpose? First, you must kneel and extend your upper body toward the ground while being a wheel. Slowly begin to roll into (towards the knees) and then roll away (away away from the knees) with your body weight to perform complex movements. It will also strengthen other muscles, such as the lower back and legs, and shoulders.

(iv) Dip stands for

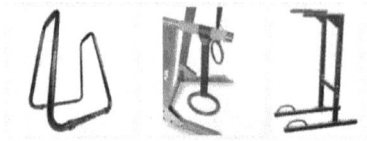

Dipping is an essential calisthenics workout for upper strength of the body.

There are two kinds of dip stands: fixed and non-fixed. They both have advantages. They are both beneficial. The difference between them is the fixed version has an adjustable width, while the other has two bars that you can adjust to your preferences.

(v) Equipment that is pushed up

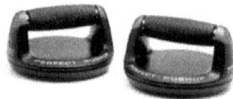

Why do you require this kind of device when you could just walk on the floor? This is because it provides additional advantages that the floor cannot. First of all, they are easy to use as they're easy to use on your wrist. Furthermore, it's easy to lower yourself using these devices. Additionally, they provide your chest an increased workout than the force it receives on the floor.

(vi) Power Towers

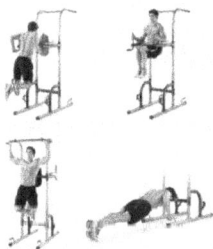

If you're looking for an all-purpose equipment that will aid you with your calisthenics workouts, then it is the best option. Find out more about its benefits below:

It lets you do both chin-ups and pull-ups for shoulders, biceps and back.

It can be used to do dip exercises to strengthen your chest.

Hanging as well as leg raising variations that will give you solid foundation.

After you've an knowledge of the equipment you can utilize and the benefits that you can get from exercises in calisthenics The next step is to examine how to begin with calisthenics. We'll discuss this in the next chapter.

Getting Started In Calisthenics

The next chapter we're going to talk about the steps to follow prior to beginning calisthenics exercises. To begin Let's look at the steps you must adhere to when beginning calisthenics exercises:

Step 1: Select an area

To ensure a properly-planned plan, you must establish a location that you'll be able for your calisthenics exercise. As people head to to work , and then go home to relax in the same manner, there should be a distinct location for your exercise. For instance, you could opt to perform your exercises in your home outside, in your backyard or even in your office , if you have the space.

Your choice will be solely based on the location you prefer to location.

STEP 2: Choose the moment to exercise at.

You must be clear on the time that you will be exercising calisthenics. This will help you stay focused and organized. There are some people who can't exercise in the morning , which is why they work out in the evening , while some exercise early in the day because they're exhausted from working. Determine which group you belong to and determine the time at which you'll be working out.

Step 3: Create your goals

In order to keep your focus on what you're doing, it is essential to begin by writing down a list of goals that you would like to attain. There are two kinds of goals, short-term and long-term. What exactly do you are looking for from calisthenics exercise in the short term , and what are the goals you are hoping to accomplish in the longer term. In this scenario you're looking to build muscle mass, but there could be other goals, such as getting rid of weight, being more fit or flexible, and a myriad of other goals. You must ensure that you have set goals that are SMART (specific achievable, measurable real-time, relevant and time-bound) goals if you truly are determined to be successful with what you're doing. In this instance the ideal short-term objective might be something like:

I will discipline myself to follow calisthenics beginner routines to get my body with the movements. Here are the routines I plan to perform every day to keep my routine daily:

Two set of push-ups with 15 repetitions, with an interval resting period of 1 minute

Two set of 10 pull-ups each with an interval resting period of one minute

Two set of 10 reps each with an interval resting period of 1 minute.

For long-term goals, you could establish goals that are SMART, such as:

My ultimate goal is to build some muscle and get a six-pack. I want to improve my leg strength and build a solid chest. To achieve this, I'll involve myself in more advanced body-training exercises. For instance:

Straight leg raises

Wide push-ups

Squat jumps

Muscle-ups

Straight bar dips

Do 3 sets of each workout each one following the next with a an interval of 20 seconds. Repeat the entire routine until exhausted.

STEP 4: Warm up

The process of warming up is of getting your muscles ready for the exercises you're going to perform. It's usually performed by stretching your arms and legs by doing simple stretches such as wrist rotations by touching your toes walking for a few minutes, and then doing arm circles.

Warm-ups allow your muscles prepare and prevent injuries, and also get the blood flowing. Another advantage is that they take only less than a minute before you're done.

STEP 5: Maintain a healthy diet

If you're looking to reap the maximum benefits the calisthenics workouts it is essential to follow a balanced diet. It can greatly assist you to renew the cells in your body and boost your energy to continue your journey. Here are a few food items you can consume:

Carbohydrates are the primary source of energy for your body. But, make sure to go for more complex carbohydrates, such as barley, brown rice and oatmeal in contrast to the easy and processed carbohydrates such as French fries, soda , etc.

Proteins contain vital amino acids that the body needs. Proteins are vital for building muscle. Some examples of foods rich in protein are eggs, fish, milk beans, nuts, and fish. In this case it is recommended to avoid eating regular consumption of red meat since it can hinder your goal.

Vegetables are among the most beneficial food items for calisthenics workouts. It is possible to eat tomatoes, spinach, kales and mushrooms.

Fruits - Fruits are an excellent source of vitamins within our bodies. They aid in replenishing our energy. Some of the fruits you can consume include watermelon, mangoes bananas, oranges, and apples.

Here's a one day menu plan you can follow to completely change your life

Day 1:

Breakfast 1

1/2 medium or small size cantaloupe

1 scoop of protein whey

2. Breakfast (about an hour following breakfast 1, above)

One cup oatmeal

Ham and cheese Ham and cheese omelet (made out of 1/4 cup cheese free of fat 2 slices of deli ham with low fat and two large eggs)

Late morning snack

1 cup of mixed berries in lower fat Greek yogurt

Lunch

1 tablespoon olive oil as well as 1 teaspoon balsamic vinegar.

2 cups mixed greens , including spinach

4 8 ounces of ground beef that is lean and lean

One whole hamburger bun made of wheat

Midday snack

Five Whole wheat crackers (try mixing mayo with the chicken and eat it on crackers

1 tablespoon light mayonnaise

3 2 ounces of canned chicken breasts

Dinner

6 8 ounces of chicken breasts

One cup of broccoli chopped

2 cups of mixed leaves (ensure that there is spinach)

1 teaspoon of balsamic vinegar, and 1 tablespoon olive oil

Nighttime snack

2.25 tablespoons of salsa (try mixing salsa with cottage cheese)

3/4 cup cottage cheese

You might be wondering why your meal program contains certain ingredients. Here's a page that will explain the ingredients that are extremely beneficial to build lean muscle.

These are only examples to help you understand the foods you can enjoy. It is now time to develop a balanced schedule based on the above categories of foods to ensure optimal growth of your muscles.

Once you've started when you begin, you must set some key things in your the mind of anyone who wants to be a pro at calisthenics. What are the things you can do to improve the chances of success exercising?

Chapter 13: Top 5 Bodyweight Exercises

In this section, I'd like to provide you with five most frequently used bodyweight exercises that can ensure outcomes. These include pushups pull ups, bodyweight bodyweight squats as well as single stiff-legged deadlifts and planks. You've likely heard of pushups pull ups, squats and planks in the past and might have attempted them but not deadlifts that are single stiff legged. I'll show you how to complete these exercises, and to fulfill the goal of creating this guide into an entire package, I will explain to you how to perform the other four exercises correctly.

Pushups

Set up for push ups

If you are lying on the ground put your hands down at a distance just a little wider than shoulder width apart.

Your feet must be set in a manner that is comfortable and feels natural to you.

Imagine your body as one huge straight line

If you're having trouble finding the right form for your body, consider the following (yes this is real)

Your eyes should be towards the future rather than straight down

When you are done with your push-up your arms should be straight and able to support your weight.

How do you finish the push up

While your arms are straight, your butt locked, and your abs braced

Do not let your elbows fly all the way to the side with every repetition.

When your chest is on the flooring (or your arms drop to 90 degrees)

Congratulations! You just completed the right push up.

Here are some alternatives to push ups to try out once you've mastered the regular push-ups to ensure an appropriate "progressive overload"

One foot push-up Do a push-up: raise one legs and then do a push up

Decline push-up: place your leg on a chair, or another place higher than the floor , and begin your push-up

The triceps (diamond) Push ups: Create the shape of a diamond using your hands. Then, begin doing push-ups using this position.

Plyometric push ups: While you are getting up after doing push-ups, press really hard to get yourself off the ground.

Clapping push-up: perform the plyometric pushup but only if you are is high enough you are able to hold your hands and clap them while you are in the air.

Pull up

Pull-ups are more simple in terms of procedure, but lots of people are having difficulty making even one pull up. Below are some steps to follow when pulling ups.

Pull up a bar using your palms facing the outside.

Lift your bodyweight so that the chin sits over the bar.

Your arms will be fully extended.

If you're not strong enough for one pull-up, I'd like to suggest you!

Start by doing dumbbell rows. strengthen your back muscles.

Implement inverted row

Place yourself on the floor beneath the bar

Hold the bar using the grip of your overhand (palms towards the side away towards you).

Engage your abs and make sure you maintain your body in a straight line.

Bring yourself up to the bar till your chest is touching the bar.

Lower yourself again.

Do a negative pull-up: reaching the bar's top and then coming down slowly and with control slowly descend.

Then, pull it all up when you're at the point of doing it!

Squat

Here's how you can do the bodyweight squat

Place your feet wide apart. It is possible to place your hands on top of your head. This is your starting point.

Start beginning by stretching your knees, and your hips. Then, sit back and relax your hips.

Continue to lower down to the maximum depth, if you're capable, then quickly reverse the movement until you get back to the starting position. While squatting make sure to keep your chest and head upwards and extend your knees forward.

Plank

Here's how to make an incline plank.

Begin by putting yourself into the press up position.

Bend your elbows and place your weight on your forearms, not your hands.

Your body should create an uniform line from your shoulders to your ankles.

Connect your abdominal muscles by suctioning your belly button towards your spine.

Keep that position during the specified duration.

Single deadlift with stiff legs

Place feet together, with hands between your thighs. Move leg up slightly until feet are not far from the floor.

Lower your torso downwards and forwards while lifting the lifted leg behind.

Keep your back straight, and the your leg's knee will bent slightly.

Keep the knee and hip of the elevated leg straight throughout the motion.

Once the stretch is felt or hands are touching the floor, return to your initial position by lifting the torso, while lowering the lifted leg.

Straighten knees of the leg that supports you when torso rises.

Repeat.

After you've learned the 5 of the best bodyweight exercises It's time to create plans and use what we've learned to get into the best shape for the year!

Chapter 14: How To Prepare Yourself Mentally For The Program

Now that you've learned a bit more about bodyweight exercise and the basic principles we'll be using throughout the course. The first thing we need to consider before we begin is the mindset we adopt.

What we need to know are the factors that are slowing us down and the best way to get past the barriers and start the process. Do you know where to begin, and you spend most of your time in search of how to do? Perhaps you've decided that you're not going to try because you're afraid of failing or feel you're not competent enough?

Most people, when they set goals for themselves never meet their goals. A majority of people, particularly when they make their New Year's Resolutions do not achieve them due to giving up within a few months of having decided to make a make a change. Whatever your age, whether you're a beginner in bodyweight training or have previous experience, we must to ensure that we're doing all we can to keep in line with the fitness objectives we have set.

5 Tips & Tricks To Stay Mentally Alert To Workout:

1 . We must begin by being present in the present moment. It's one of the best things we could accomplish to overcome any resistance we may have to the things we'd like to accomplish and also have a clear idea of what we want to do, but aren't sure how to go about it. There are a myriad of methods to get present, however one of the most popular options is "Mindful Meditation".

A few examples of Mindful Meditation could include a practice where the person focuses on sitting and observing the moment. It's a blend with deep breaths, relaxation, and paying attention to being present in the moment. It's about taking action to take you out of your mind. In order to be present, you don't need to be meditative even though it's among the best methods to be present.

You are free to do what you like if it helps get you off your feet. You could have a passion that you enjoy, it might be taking walking, dancing or even swimming. Make a habit that allows you to become more present in order to make more progress towards your objectives.

2. It is important to identify what we are looking for in our fitness goals. We require a compelling justification for the reason we're seeking it. It's not going to suffice to

say that I'd like to be in excellent shape and have abs that are six-pack. This is more of a wishful-thinking attitude. For instance, if you would like to get six-pack abs, you must you must find a more compelling reason or motive in order to attain it, but make it more precise. For instance:

"I'll achieve my dream physique and have the body I've always wanted since I'm looking to be beautiful and healthy. I would like to look more attractive to men of other sex and be a source of inspiration for others by the incredible outcomes I'll achieve. I'll have a lot of energy and be filled with excitement and vitality I can't wait to begin working towards my dream"'

No matter what our motivation is to get healthy and fit it is essential to be driven by a passion to be motivated to work towards your fitness objectives. If we don't have a solid motivation and the desire to achieve our goals, then there's no sense in setting objectives because you'll give up after three days or even one week.

3. It is imperative to perform all things to our best ability. At first it's possible that we don't know all we are able to do but it's all just an ongoing process, and it's crucial that to treat it that way and not let ourselves become discouraged.

As we begin our journey, we may not be in the form we'd like to be in our training, especially if it's about our body or our performance in athletics. These kinds of things could cause us to feel down. Do not make comparisons to other people who have expertise ahead of you and it's not a fair one to draw. Concentrate on your goals and begin there. It's as easy as it gets.

4. We must be aware that we have the power to make changes, nobody else does other than you. You can't count on anyone else to change us, because the reality is that no one can change unless they wish to regardless of what other people tell them.

We must be in alignment with the goals and aspirations in our lives and set goals and plans for achieving these goals. We should be more self-centered regarding what we would like instead of having others taking our decisions.

5. The last but not least the fact that we should never quit. Naturally, life will sometimes interfere of our goals and we may skip a workout or begin to make excuses as reasons why we're unable to exercise on the day. The most important thing to keep in mind is the ultimate goal that we set to ourselves. This is why, once

we've established our fitness goals , we have to record it on the paper and put it somewhere where you is always visible.

There must be the environment around us which always remind us of our goals and the physique we wish to attain. It might be your training journal or someone you admire and admire. Whatever the case, we must remind ourselves of our ultimate goal.

Set Up The Right Diet Plan & Get Started

After we've identified our goals and purpose with our training, we must ensure that we have the correct program for our diet too. Because , let's face the facts that we'll never get anywhere without a solid nutrition plan. In this article, I'll provide you with a few basic actions you can take to make sure you have a particular diet plan that is tailored to your needs.

The diet and fitness arena is a large subject as there are hundreds of thousands of regimens and diets that individuals use based the goals they have set for themselves. In the majority of optionsavailable it's difficult to figure out where to begin.

I believe that lots of people make it more complicated and difficult than it already is and that's not what it should be. Dieting isn't a difficult issue that has to be your second job or even your new six-year education from your college.

There are tricks and tips that can be used to make dieting simpler and enjoyable. I'll show you how how to accomplish this too. There is no need to count calories. We don't need the burden of weighing our meals items, we don't need to learn things about macros, and we don't need to buy a fridge that holds all our food items.

Nothing of this are we required to know. It is possible to simplify things and still be efficient.

Since, let's face it that we're ordinary guys. We're sure not looking forward to running naked in front of a crowd to display our accomplishments. This is something for the serious bodybuilders to compete in. Some of the fitness experts may even offer others fitness tips about the latest apps they can use to track their calories. They say that by snapping a photo of their meals, the app will calculate calories of their food for them. It's a fact do you truly think that your calorie-counting app is trustworthy by taking a photo of food items?

This is similar to me claiming having an application that, by taking a photo of you, I will be able to determine your body weight, fat-percentage or your IQ. Maybe even the amount of time you're going to McDonald's. It's just ridiculous.

It's not my intention to say that one is better than the other. What am I saying is that something that works great for one person may not be a good fit for someone else.

People who aren't taking bodybuilding as a part of their lifestyle may not want to take this kind of extreme diet and nutrition program.

The most simple and effective method is known as "The Portion Size Method". There's no doubt that it can be described in many different names, and is utilized by many people in the industry of fitness. This method will make losing weight more simple, and the most appealing aspect of this strategy is the fact that all that you require is a plate that can be used to separate your meals throughout the day.

It's not necessary to have a useless app that snaps pictures of your food items to determine the amount of calories you've consumed.

Use a dinner-sized plate to divide the the plate into two. The left-hand side fill the plate with protein while on the other side, you will fill the plate with carbs. It's as simple as that. When it comes to vegetables, based on whether you're cutting or bulking, make the same preparation. Divide the the plate in two , and on the left you will find your protein and on the other side the vegetables.

Here's an example of what your eating habits during the day with the method of portion size:

Sample Meal Plan For Someone Trying To Gain Muscle

7:15 a.m. Protein, Carb, or Fruit

9:30 a.m Protein, Carb or Fruit

12:30 am Protein, Carb or Fruit

22:30 p.m. Protein, Carb or Fruit

5:30 p.m. Protein, Carb or Fruit

7:15 p.m. Protein, Vegetables

Sample Meal Plan For Someone Trying To Lose Fat

(if you're trying to shed weight, cut off all carbs and eat only Protein vegetables, Protein, and fruits.

7:15 a.m. Protein, Vegetables or Fruit

9:30 a.m Protein, Vegetables or Fruit

12:30 am Protein, Vegetables or Fruit

22:30 p.m. Protein, Vegetables or Fruit

5:30 p.m. Protein, Vegetables or Fruit

7:15 p.m. Protein, Vegetables or Fruit

Example Meal Plan for Those Trying to gain muscle mass and lose fat simultaneously.

7:15 a.m. Protein, Carb, or Fruit

9:30 a.m Protein, Carb or Fruit

12:30 am Protein, Carb or Fruit

2.30 p.m. Protein, Vegetables

5:30 p.m. Protein, Vegetables

7:15 p.m. Protein, Vegetables

Food Choices

Proteins

Fish

Chicken

Lean Steak

Lean Ham

Tuna

Salmon

Whole Eggs

CARBOHYDRATES

Brown Rice

Wild Rice

Wheat Pasta

Oatmeal

Beans

Sweet Potatoes

VEGETABLES

Broccoli

Snow Peas

Peppers

Lettuce

Eggplant

String Beans

Spinach

Cucumbers

FRUITS

Any fruit that isn't canned is excellent

It is not necessary to follow this schedule like you are a slave. If the schedule isn't a good fit for you Simply modify and alter the schedule to suit your needs. It's as easy as that.

Chapter 15: Simple, Easy And Effective Exercises For Beginners

Exercise for Beginners

Don't be discouraged even if it will be the first time you're physically active. Everybody has to begin somewhere. Another aspect you need to keep in mind is that your path will include both positive and negative elements. It is possible to see weeks and days pass with significant progress and gains. You may also observe other periods of time in which there doesn't seem to be any significant change.

It is scientifically proven how the body functions. In the beginning you'll see rapid changes, but you could begin to experience the plateau appear after a couple of months. This simply means that you should keep working hard. This means that you have built up enough strength that your previous workouts aren't sufficient anymore. Score!

Keep on track and maintain a positive attitude. There is no way to be wrong with a regular vigorous exercise, along with a healthy and balanced diet.

If you're unfamiliar with calisthenics or fitness in general, you can rest sure that there is many exercises you can try to get a slimmer body. From squats and push-ups, you can do any of these workouts anywhere.

Be aware that prior to participating in any form of strenuous exercise, ensure that you talk to a physician. It is crucial to have a medical clearance for physical activity in order to lower the chance of injuries.

Types of Exercises

Here are a few of the most commonly used and simple exercises that you can begin incorporating into your routine. It is possible to begin by performing anywhere from 10 to 20 repetitions of each exercise, for the total of 4 sets.

One way to figure out the number of reps needed for an ideal workout is to the halfway mark on reps. When you are around halfway through, it will begin to feel difficult, but not so difficult that you can't complete the set. This will be your method to determine how many reps you'll be able to do within the course of a set.

PUSH-UPS

Take a step forward standing on your feet. Maintain your palms on the floor, and your toes parallel towards the ground. Make sure you keep your core firm and let your body remain in line with the floor.

Slowly, begin to lower your chest toward the floor and then extend your elbows.

Re-inforce your body by to bring yourself to return to the plank position.

Reverse the exercise and repeat the reps until you've completed them.

JUMPING JACKS

From the beginning in the beginning, stand straight and tall, with your feet together, and your arms at your sides.

When you leap with your feet towards your sides, swiftly lift your arms above your head.

After that, jump to your seated position then bring your arms to your sides.

Repeat the steps until you have completed your set.

SQUATS

Place your feet on the ground , with your feet approximately shoulder width apart, looking toward the forward direction with your shoulder-length pulled away.

Spread your arms out in front of you so that they are close to the floor. This will assist you in maintaining your stability.

Reduce your body to the point that you were sitting in the chair. Keep your chin upwards while you move your upper body toward the side. Let your back bend slightly while keeping your chest in place.

When you are squatting your thighs should be in line with the floor. Be sure to put your your heels to prevent your knees from passing the front of your toes.

Engage your core muscles and get yourself back to the starting point. Make sure that you keep the weight distribution within your heels.

Repeat steps to complete your set.

CHAIR DIPS

Find a sturdy bench or bench, and sit in front of it , facing towards the back of your seat.

Place your feet on the edge of your seat and put your hands between your hips. Your palms should be at the edge, and the shoulders must be centered.

Get off the chair and walk a little forward until you're able to no longer be seated on the chair.

Hold your body in place with your hands. Keep your head and chest up , and your keep your core engaged.

Bring your body toward the floor slowly, but make sure that your elbows are not allowed to reach at a 90-degree angle.

Reach your arms out and raise your body up using your triceps back to the position you started from.

Repeat steps to complete your set.

SIT-UPS

Find a spot to lie in a position that is flat across your back. It is suggested to choose the floor to be somewhat soft to ensure that you don't put too much pressure on your back.

Make a slight bend in your knees, then place your heels onto the flooring.

Based on your personal preference, what feels your comfort level, put your hands on your head or place your arms over your chest.

Close your core and make sure that your core is fully active all the time.

Slowly sit up while maintaining your chin up and your feet firmly to the ground.

Your chest should touch your knees.

Slowly lower yourself to your starting point.

Continue to follow the steps to complete your set.

Complete 4 sets of each of these calisthenics workouts can aid in increasing your endurance and strength.

As time passes, you will be able to increase the amount of repetitions and resistance as you progress through your training. You can add variations on the exercises in order to increase the difficulty for you.

In the near future, you'll be able to increase in intensity and include advanced forms of exercise.

Chapter 16: Bodybuilding Exercises For Beginners

Below are some tips to think about prior to starting an exercise routine.

Be bold, but be the basics in mind:

I'm not trying claim that you shouldn't build large muscles, but you must establish your primary goal for yourself, and make sure they can be achieved and assessed. There's no sense to set a goal that is beyond reach and could result in negative results. Consider what you would like to achieve in the next few months, take a look at your current circumstances and strengths and set realistic goals in this respect. Additionally, consider the long term, and think about what your final outcome will appear to be. Utilize your short-term goals to guarantee the long-term success of your business.

Do not expect to see results overnight.

It is common to see results rapidly. It is essential to complete a long period of work before analysing the outcomes. A lot of people will be in the position they'd like to be within only a couple of weeks, but it's usually more difficult.Keep in your mind that you'll shape your body with time and your future goals will be attained if you maintain. With your objectives in mind and you're thinking right we can examine a specific workout.

For a beginner to the field of bodybuilding and development it is recommended to do 15 exercises that are based on basic movements that involve different muscles simultaneously. It will help to have the exercises in a set of repetitions in groups and regularly mix them up to ensure your body is not used to the movements you desire. Training 3 times per week for 3 months or more. The best exercises to perform simultaneously with different muscle groups, like squats, bench presses and pulls.Before every session, you should get your body ready for the workout with 10 minutes of basic aerobic exerciselike cycling, walking, running and resting. Are you sweating already? It's because your body isn't well-equipped for the toughest workouts you'll need to perform to increase muscle mass.

Set, repeat, and rest

Start slowly in the initial month of your training, and remain focused. Do various exercises, with between 15 and 20 repetitions per Minute. The weight will be increased and increased during each exercise. You should rest for 30 to 40 minutes between sets. Also, increase your weight slightly in every workout.This can prevent your muscles from working too hard.

Conclusion

I hope that this book is useful in helping you to learn about calisthenics and the benefits of specific exercises, and the main reasons you should take on an exercise routine that incorporates calisthenics. I hope that you enjoyed the list of diverse calisthenics exercises. With clear instructions, you will be able to quickly comprehend both the standard exercises, and the more obscure ones.

It is the next stage to develop your own calisthenics exercise plan. Because this book has discussion on the development of your own fitness program, you will be able to combine all the lessons, make an outline, and count on it to start doing your workouts according to plan.